ANTI AGING JUICING AND SMOOTHIES

Healthy and Delicious fruit juice to promote longevity and make you look younger

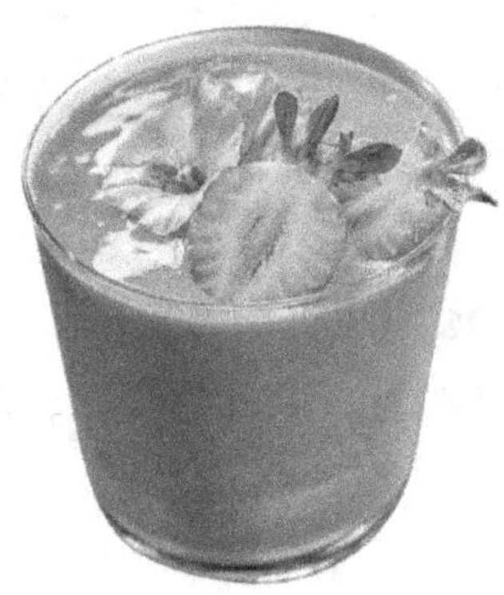

Dr. Malvin harison

TABLE OF CONTENT

Introduction

Welcome to the world of juicing, where nature's vibrant bounty combines with the power of antioxidants to create a potent elixir for anti-aging. In this beginner's guide, we present 30 rejuvenating juicing recipes that will help nourish your body, enhance your skin's radiance, and promote overall vitality.

Each recipe is carefully crafted with ingredients specifically chosen for their anti-aging properties. So, grab your juicer, prepare your taste buds, and embark on a transformative journey to embrace the fountain of youth.

Importance of anti aging juicing and smoothie for beginners

Anti-aging juicing and smoothies for beginners hold significant importance in fostering overall well-being and vitality. Here are key reasons why incorporating these beverages into a beginner's routine can be beneficial:

1. Nutrient-Rich Boost: Juicing and smoothies offer a convenient and efficient way to consume a concentrated dose of essential nutrients, including vitamins, minerals, antioxidants, and phytochemicals. These nutrients are crucial for cellular health, skin rejuvenation, and overall bodily functions.

2. Hydration Reinforcement: Many fruits and vegetables used in juicing and smoothies have high water content, contributing to hydration.

3. Digestive Health: Fiber-rich fruits and vegetables in smoothies contribute to digestive health. Fiber aids in digestion, supports gut microbiota, and helps prevent issues like constipation.

4. Reduced Inflammation: Anti-inflammatory compounds present in certain ingredients, such as berries and leafy greens, may help reduce inflammation in the body.

5. Cellular Repair and Protection: Antioxidants found in fruits and vegetables combat oxidative stress, protecting cells from damage and supporting the body's natural processes of repair and regeneration.

6. Energy Boost: The natural sugars in fruits provide a quick energy boost, while the fiber helps sustain energy levels over time. This can be particularly beneficial for beginners who are looking to improve their energy and stamina.

7. Weight Management: Including nutrient-dense, low-calorie ingredients in juicing and smoothies can be part of a balanced approach to weight management, helping beginners achieve and maintain a healthy weight.

8. Simple Incorporation of Superfoods: Juicing and smoothies provide an easy way to incorporate superfoods like chia seeds, flaxseeds, or spirulina, which are rich in nutrients and known for their potential health benefits.

9. Easy Adaptation for Beginners: For those new to a healthy lifestyle, juicing and smoothies offer a palatable and enjoyable way to introduce more fruits and vegetables into their diet. It's a beginner-friendly approach to embracing a nutrient-rich lifestyle.

10. Customization and Variety: Beginners can experiment with different fruits, vegetables, and add-ins to tailor their juicing and smoothie experience. This versatility ensures a variety of flavors and nutritional profiles.

In summary, anti-aging juicing and smoothies provide a convenient and enjoyable avenue for beginners to access a powerhouse of nutrients. As a delicious and healthful addition to one's routine, these beverages contribute to overall health, energy, and the pursuit of a vibrant, age-defying lifestyle.

Chapter 1: Anti Aging Juices For Beginners

Here are 30 Juicing for Anti-Aging Recipes: A Beginner's Guide to Radiant Health

1. Green Goddess Glow

Ingredients

- 2 cups spinach
- 1 cucumber
- 1 green apple
- 1 lemon (peeled)
- 1-inch piece of ginger

Instructions

1. Wash all the ingredients thoroughly.
2. Chop the cucumber, apple, and ginger into manageable pieces.
3. Add the spinach, cucumber, apple, lemon, and ginger to your juicer.
4. Juice the ingredients until well blended.

5. Pour the juice into a glass, stir gently, and enjoy the refreshing taste of youthful radiance.

2. Berry Blast of Antioxidants

Ingredients

- 1 cup mixed berries (strawberries, blueberries, raspberries)
- 1 ripe banana
- 1 cup coconut water
- 1 tablespoon chia seeds

Instructions

1. Wash the berries and remove any stems.
2. Peel and slice the banana.
3. Add the berries, banana, coconut water, and chia seeds to your juicer.
4. Juice the ingredients until smooth.
5. Pour the juice into a glass, give it a quick stir, and relish in the antioxidant-rich goodness.

3. Citrus Zing Revitalizer

Ingredients

- 2 oranges (peeled)
- 2 carrots
- 1-inch piece of turmeric root
- 1 tablespoon honey (optional)

Instructions

1. Peel the oranges and chop them into quarters.
2. Wash and chop the carrots into manageable pieces.
3. Peel the turmeric root.
4. Add the oranges, carrots, turmeric root, and honey (if desired) to your juicer.
5. Juice the ingredients until well combined.
6. Pour the juice into a glass, give it a gentle stir, and savor the invigorating zing of citrus.

4. Tropical Glow

Ingredients
- 1 cup pineapple chunks
- 1 mango (peeled and pitted)
- 1 kiwi (peeled)
- 1 cup coconut water

Instructions
1. Cut the pineapple, mango, and kiwi into manageable pieces.
2. Add the pineapple, mango, kiwi, and coconut water to your juicer.
3. Juice the ingredients until smooth.
4. Pour the juice into a glass, stir gently, and enjoy the tropical flavors of youthful radiance.

5. Beetroot Beauty

Ingredients
- 1 beetroot (peeled)
- 2 carrots
- 1 orange (peeled)
- 1-inch piece of ginger

Instructions

1. Wash and chop the beetroot, carrots, and ginger.
2. Peel the orange and separate it into segments.
3. Add the beetroot, carrots, orange segments, and ginger to your juicer.
4. Juice the ingredients until well blended.
5. Pour the juice into a glass, give it a quick stir, and savor the earthy sweetness of this beauty-enhancing concoction.

6. Green Detoxifier

Ingredients

- 2 cups kale
- 1 cucumber
- 2 green apples
- 1 lemon (peeled)
- 1 stalk celery

Instructions

1. Wash all the ingredients thoroughly.
2. Chop the cucumber, apples, and celery into manageable pieces.

3. Add the kale, cucumber, apples, lemon, and celery to your juicer.

4. Juice the ingredients until well combined.

5. Pour the juice into a glass, stir gently, and enjoy the detoxifying freshness.

7. Carrot-Citrus Refresher

Ingredients

- 4 carrots
- 2 oranges (peeled)
- 1 lemon (peeled)
- 1-inch piece of ginger

Instructions

1. Wash and chop the carrots into manageable pieces.

2. Peel the oranges and lemon, and separate them into segments.

3. Peel the ginger.

4. Add the carrots, oranges, lemon segments, and ginger to your juicer.

5. Juice the ingredients until well blended.

6. Pour the juice into a glass, give it a quick stir, and relish in the revitalizing citrus burst.

8. Pomegranate Power

Ingredients:
- 1 cup pomegranate seeds
- 1 apple
- 1 cucumber
- 1 lime (peeled)
- A handful of mint leaves

Instructions

1. Wash and deseed the pomegranate.

2. Chop the apple and cucumber into manageable pieces.

3. Add the pomegranate seeds, apple, cucumber, lime, and mint leaves to your juicer.

4. Juice the ingredients until smooth.

5. Pour the juice into a glass, stir gently, and embrace the refreshing power of pomegranate.

9. Blueberry Bliss

Ingredients:
- 1 cup blueberries
- 1 banana
- 1 cup almond milk
- 1 tablespoon flax seeds

Instructions

1. Wash the blueberries.
2. Peel and slice the banana.
3. Add the blueberries, banana, almond milk, and flaxseeds to your juicer.
4. Juice the ingredients until well combined.
5. Pour the juice into a glass, give it a gentle stir, and relish in the antioxidant-rich bliss.

10. Gingered Greens

Ingredients
- 2 cups spinach
- 1 green apple
- 1 cucumber
- 1 lemon (peeled)
- 1-inch piece of ginger

Instructions

1. Wash all the ingredients thoroughly.

2. Chop the apple, cucumber, and ginger into manageable pieces.

3. Add the spinach, apple, cucumber, lemon, and ginger to your juicer.

4. Juice the ingredients until well blended.

5. Pour the juice into a glass, stir gently, and enjoy the invigorating combination of greens and ginger.

11. Watermelon Refresher

Ingredients:

- 2 cups watermelon (seedless)
- 1 lime (peeled)
- A handful of fresh mint leaves

Instructions:

1. Cut the watermelon into cubes, removing any seeds.

2. Peel the lime.

3. Add the watermelon, lime, and mint leaves to your juicer.

4. Juice the ingredients until smooth.

5. Pour the juice into a glass, give it a quick stir, and savor the hydrating and cooling effect of this refreshing concoction.

12. Cabbage Cleanser

Ingredients
- 2 cups purple cabbage
- 2 green apples
- 1 lemon (peeled)
- 1-inch piece of ginger

Instructions
1. Wash the cabbage and chop it into manageable pieces.
2. Chop the apples and ginger into manageable pieces.
3. Ground all the ingredients together and add the lemon juice.
4. Serve chilled

13. Pineapple Papaya Punch

Ingredients:
- 1 cup pineapple chunks
- 1 cup papaya chunks

- 1 orange (peeled)
- 1-inch piece of turmeric root

Instructions

1. Cut the pineapple and papaya into chunks.

2. Peel the orange and separate it into segments.

3. Peel the turmeric root.

4. Add the pineapple, papaya, orange segments, and turmeric root to your juicer.

5. Juice the ingredients until well combined.

6. Pour the juice into a glass, stir gently, and enjoy the tropical flavors of this refreshing punch.

14. Kale-Cucumber Cooler

Ingredients:
- 2 cups kale
- 1 cucumber
- 1 green apple
- 1 lime (peeled)
- A handful of fresh mint leaves

Instructions

1. Wash all the ingredients thoroughly.

2. Chop the cucumber and apple into manageable pieces.

3. Add the kale, cucumber, apple, lime, and mint leaves to your juicer.

4. Juice the ingredients until well blended.

5. Pour the juice into a glass, stir gently, and relish in the cooling and invigorating properties of this green concoction.

15. Carrot-Orange Sunrise

Ingredients:

- 4 carrots
- 2 oranges (peeled)
- 1-inch piece of ginger
- 1 tablespoon honey (optional)

Instructions

1. Wash and chop the carrots into manageable pieces.

2. Scoop the oranges and separate them into segments.

3. Peel the ginger.

4. Add the carrots, orange segments, ginger, and honey (if desired) to your juicer.

5. Juice the ingredients until well combined.

6. Pour the juice into a glass, give it a quick stir, and savor the vibrant and energizing sunrise in a glass.

16. Spinach-Berry Blast

Ingredients

- 2 cups spinach
- 1 cup mixed berries (strawberries, blueberries, raspberries)
- 1 banana
- 1 cup almond milk

Instructions

1. Wash the spinach and berries.

2. Peel and slice the banana.

3. Add the spinach, berries, banana, and almond milk to your juicer.

4. Juice the ingredients until smooth.

5. Pour the juice into a glass, give it a gentle stir, and enjoy the antioxidant-rich burst of flavors.

17. Turmeric-Ginger Tonic

Ingredients:
- 1 orange (peeled)
- 1 lemon (peeled)
- 1-inch piece of turmeric root
- 1-inch piece of ginger
- 1 tablespoon honey (optional)

Instructions

1. Peel the orange and lemon, and separate them into segments.
2. Peel the turmeric root and ginger.
3. Add the orange segments, lemon segments, turmeric root, ginger, and honey (if desired) to your juicer.
4. Juice the ingredients until well blended.
5. Pour the juice into a glass, give it a quick stir, and savor the immune-boosting and anti-inflammatory properties of this tonic.

18. Mango-Green Tea Refresher

Ingredients:

- 1 cup mango chunks
- 1 green tea bag (brewed and cooled)
- 1 lime (peeled)
- A handful of fresh mint leaves

Instructions:

1. Cut the mango into chunks.
2. Brew green tea and let it cool.
3. Peel the lime.
4. Add the mango chunks, cooled green tea, lime, and mint leaves to your juicer.
5. Juice the ingredients until smooth.
6. Pour the juice into a glass, stir gently, and enjoy the tropical flavors with a refreshing twist of green tea.

19. Cucumber-Melon Hydrator

Ingredients:

- 1 cucumber
- 1 cup honeydew melon chunks
- 1 cup watermelon chunks
- 1 lime (peeled)

Instructions:

1. Wash and chop the cucumber into manageable pieces.

2. Cut the honeydew melon and watermelon into chunks.

3. Peel the lime.

4. Add the cucumber, honeydew melon chunks, watermelon chunks, and lime to your juicer.

5. Juice the ingredients until well combined.

6. Pour the juice into a glass, give it a quick stir, and savor the hydrating and cooling effect of this refreshing elixir.

20. Green Goddess Elixir

Ingredients

- 2 cups spinach
- 1 green apple
- 1 cucumber
- 1 lime (peeled)
- 1 tablespoon spirulina powder (optional)

Instructions

1. Wash all the ingredients thoroughly.

2. Chop the apple and cucumber into manageable pieces.

3. Peel the lime.

4. Add the spinach, apple, cucumber, lime, and spirulina powder (if using) to your juicer.

5. Juice the ingredients until well blended.

6. Pour the juice into a glass, stir gently, and enjoy the refreshing and detoxifying effects of this green elixir.

21. Citrus-Carrot Glow

Ingredients

- 4 carrots
- 2 oranges (peeled)
- 1 grapefruit (peeled)
- 1-inch piece of ginger

Instructions

1. Wash and chop the carrots into manageable pieces.

2. Peel the oranges and grapefruit, and separate them into segments.

3. Peel the ginger.

4. Add the carrots, orange segments, grapefruit segments, and ginger to your juicer.

5. Juice the ingredients until well blended.

6. Pour the juice into a glass, give it a quick stir, and enjoy the vitamin C-rich glow.

22. Kale-Pineapple Detox

Ingredients

- 2 cups kale
- 1 cup pineapple chunks
- 1 cucumber
- 1 lemon (peeled)

Instructions

1. Wash all the ingredients thoroughly.

2. Chop the pineapple and cucumber into manageable pieces.

3. Add the kale, pineapple chunks, cucumber, and lemon to your juicer.

4. Juice the ingredients until well combined.

5. Pour the juice into a glass, stir gently, and embrace the detoxifying and refreshing properties of this green elixir.

23. Apple-Celery Refresher

Ingredients

- 2 green apples
- 2 stalks celery
- 1 lemon (peeled)
- A handful of fresh parsley

Instructions

1. Wash all the ingredients thoroughly.
2. Chop the apples and celery into manageable pieces.
3. Peel the lemon.
4. Add the apples, celery, lemon, and parsley to your juicer.
5. Juice the ingredients until well blended.
6. Pour the juice into a glass, give it a quick stir, and enjoy the crisp and rejuvenating flavors.

24. Cucumber-Mint Cooler

Ingredients:

- 2 cucumbers
- A handful of fresh mint leaves

- 1 lime (peeled)
- 1 tablespoon honey (optional)

Instructions

1. Wash the cucumbers and mint leaves.
2. Chop the cucumbers into manageable pieces.
3. Peel the lime.
4. Add the cucumbers, mint leaves, lime, and honey (if desired) to your juicer.
5. Juice the ingredients until well combined.
6. Pour the juice into a glass, give it a quick stir, and relish in the cooling and refreshing effect of this revitalizing cooler.

25. Watermelon-Basil Quencher

Ingredients

- 2 cups watermelon (seedless)
- A handful of fresh basil leaves
- 1 lime (peeled)

Instructions

1. Cut the watermelon into cubes, removing any seeds.
2. Wash the basil leaves.
3. Peel the lime.
4. Add the watermelon cubes, basil leaves, and lime to your juicer.
5. Juice the ingredients until smooth.
6. Pour the juice into a glass, stir gently, and enjoy the hydrating and rejuvenating properties of this delightful quencher.

26. Mango-Coconut Delight

Ingredients

- 1 cup mango chunks
- 1 cup coconut water
- 1 banana
- 1 tablespoon chia seeds

Instructions

1. Cut the mango into chunks.

2. Peel and slice the banana.

3. Add the mango chunks, coconut water, banana, and chia seeds to your juicer.

4. Juice the ingredients until well combined.

5. Pour the juice into a glass, give it a gentle stir, and indulge in the tropical flavors and nourishing benefits.

27. Spinach-Pineapple Reviver

Ingredients

- 2 cups spinach
- 1 cup pineapple chunks
- 1 green apple
- 1 lemon (peeled)
- 1-inch piece of ginger

Instructions

1. Wash all the ingredients thoroughly.

2. Chop the pineapple and apple into manageable pieces.

3. Add the spinach, pineapple chunks, apple, lemon, and ginger to your juicer.

4. Juice the ingredients until well blended.

5. Pour the juice into a glass, stir gently, and embrace the revitalizing and rejuvenating essence of this green reviver.

28. Blueberry-Beet Booster

Ingredients

- 1 cup blueberries
- 1 beetroot (peeled)
- 1 orange (peeled)
- 1 tablespoon flax seeds

Instructions

1. Wash the blueberries.

2. Chop the beetroot into manageable pieces.

3. Peel the orange and separate it into segments.

4. Add the blueberries, beetroot, orange segments, and flaxseeds to your juicer.

5. Juice the ingredients until well combined.

6. Pour the juice into a glass, give it a quick stir, and enjoy the antioxidant-rich boost of flavors.

29. Pomegranate-Grape Elixir

Ingredients

- 1 cup pomegranate arils
- 1 cup red grapes
- 1 lemon (peeled)
- A handful of fresh mint leaves

Instructions

1. Wash the pomegranate arils and grapes.
2. Peel the lemon.
3. Add the pomegranate arils, grapes, lemon, and mint leaves to your juicer.
4. Juice the ingredients until well blended.
5. Pour the juice into a glass, stir gently, and savor the vibrant and refreshing elixir.

30. Carrot-Beet Radiance

Ingredients

- 4 carrots
- 1 beetroot (peeled)
- 1 orange (peeled)
- 1-inch piece of ginger

Instructions

1. Wash and chop the carrots into manageable pieces.

2. Chop the beetroot into manageable pieces.

3. Peel the orange and separate it into segments.

4. Peel the ginger.

5. Add the carrots, beetroot, orange segments, and ginger to your juicer.

6. Juice the ingredients until well combined.

7. Pour the juice into a glass, give it a quick stir, and embrace the radiant and nourishing properties of this vibrant blend.

Chapter 2: Anti Aging Smoothie For Beginners

Here are smoothie recipes that incorporate ingredients known for their anti-aging properties:

1. Berry Blast

Ingredients
- 1 cup of different berries (blueberries, raspberries, strawberries)
- 1/2 cup spinach
- 1/2 cup almond milk
- 1 tablespoon chia seeds
- 1 teaspoon honey (optional)
- Ice cubes (optional)

Instructions: Blend all the ingredients until smooth and enjoy. Berries are rich in antioxidants, which help fight free radicals and reduce signs of aging.

2. Green Goddess

Ingredients

- 1 cup kale
- 1/2 cucumber
- 1/2 avocado
- 1/2 cup coconut water
- 1 tablespoon flax seeds
- Juice of 1 lemon

Instructions: Blend all the ingredients until smooth. This smoothie is packed with greens and healthy fats from avocado, which can promote youthful-looking skin.

3. Tropical Glow

Ingredients
- 1 cup pineapple chunks
- 1/2 banana
- 1/2 cup coconut milk
- 1/4 cup Greek yogurt
- 1 tablespoon coconut oil
- Handful of spinach

Instructions: Blend all the ingredients until smooth. Pineapple is rich in vitamin C, which supports collagen production and helps maintain skin elasticity.

4. Golden Elixir

Ingredients
- 1 cup almond milk
- 1/2 cup mango chunks
- 1/2 teaspoon turmeric powder
- 1/2 teaspoon ginger powder
- 1 tablespoon almond butter
- 1 teaspoon honey (optional)
- Ice cubes (optional)

Instructions: Blend all the ingredients until smooth. Turmeric and ginger have powerful anti-inflammatory properties and can help reduce signs of aging.

5. Chocolate Delight

Ingredients
- 1 cup unsweetened almond milk
- 1/2 ripe banana
- 2 tablespoons raw cacao powder
- 1 tablespoon almond butter
- 1 tablespoon honey (optional)
- Ice cubes (optional)

Instructions: Blend all the ingredients until smooth. Raw cacao is rich in antioxidants, which can help protect the skin against oxidative stress and premature aging.

6. Green Goddess Glow

Ingredients
- 1 cup spinach
- 1/2 cucumber
- 1/2 avocado
- 1/2 cup coconut water
- 1/2 cup pineapple chunks
- 1 tablespoon chia seeds

Instructions: Add all the ingredients into a blender. Blend until smooth and creamy. Pour into a glass and enjoy!

7. Berry Beauty Blast

Ingredients
- 1 cup of different berries (blueberries, strawberries)
- 1/2 cup almond milk
- 1/4 cup Greek yogurt
- 1 tablespoon honey
- 1/4 teaspoon cinnamon

Instructions: Add all the ingredients into a blender. Blend until smooth and creamy. Pour into a glass and enjoy!

8. Turmeric Tonic

Ingredients
- 1 cup unsweetened almond milk
- 1 ripe banana
- 1/2 teaspoon turmeric powder
- 1/2 teaspoon ginger powder
- 1 tablespoon almond butter
- 1 tablespoon honey

Instructions: Add all the ingredients into a blender. Blend until smooth and creamy. If desired, add ice cubes for a colder and thicker consistency. Pour into a glass and enjoy!

9. Papaya Perfection

Ingredients
- 1 cup fresh papaya chunks
- 1/2 cup coconut milk
- 1/4 cup orange juice

- 1 tablespoon flaxseed meal
- 1 tablespoon lime juice
- 1 teaspoon honey

Instructions: Add all the ingredients into a blender. Blend until smooth and creamy. If desired, add ice cubes for a colder and thicker consistency. Pour into a glass and enjoy!

10. Cocoa Collagen Crush

Ingredients

- 1 cup unsweetened almond milk
- 1/2 cup brewed green tea, chilled
- 1 tablespoon cocoa powder
- 1 scoop collagen powder
- 1/2 frozen banana
- 1 tablespoon almond butter

Instructions: Add all the ingredients into a blender. Blend until smooth and creamy. If desired, add ice cubes for a colder and thicker consistency. Pour into a glass and enjoy!

11. Kale-Banana Powerhouse

Ingredients

- 2 cups kale leaves (stems removed)
- 1 ripe banana
- 1 cup unsweetened almond milk
- 1 tablespoon almond butter
- 1 tablespoon honey (optional)

Instructions: Blend all the recipes together till smooth and creamy. Adjust the sweetness as desired.

12. Mango-Coconut Refresher:

Ingredients

- 1 ripe mango
- 1/2 cup coconut water
- 1/2 cup Greek yogurt
- 1 tablespoon shredded coconut
- 1 teaspoon lime juice

Instructions: Blend all the ingredients until well combined.

13. Spinach-Berry Antioxidant

Ingredients

- 2 cups spinach

- 1 cup mixed berries (strawberries, blueberries, raspberries)
- 1/2 cup unsweetened almond milk
- 1 tablespoon flax seeds
- 1 tablespoon honey (optional)
Instructions: Blend all the ingredients until well mixed.

14. Turmeric-Ginger Zinger

Ingredients
- 1 cup pineapple chunks
- 1/2 teaspoon turmeric powder
- 1/2 teaspoon ginger powder (or 1-inch piece of fresh ginger)
- 1 cup coconut water
- 1 tablespoon honey (optional)
Instructions: Blend all the ingredients until well combined.

15. Berry-Beet Energizer

Ingredients
- 1 cup of different berries (strawberries, blueberries, raspberries)

- 1 small beet (peeled and chopped)
- 1/2 cup unsweetened almond milk
- 1 tablespoon almond butter
- 1 tablespoon honey (optional)

Instructions: Blend all the recipes together until well combined, smooth and creamy.

16. Banana-Oat Powerhouse

Ingredients

- 1 ripe banana
- 1/2 cup rolled oats
- 1 cup unsweetened almond milk
- 1 tablespoon almond butter
- 1 teaspoon honey (optional)

Instructions: Blend all the ingredients until smooth and creamy. If desired, you can soak the oats in almond milk for a few minutes before blending to soften them.

17. Cherry-Almond Delight

Ingredients

- 1 cup cherries (pitted)

- 1 cup unsweetened almond milk
- 1 tablespoon almond butter
- 1 tablespoon honey (optional)
- A handful of ice cubes

Instructions: Blend all the ingredients together until well combined. Adjust the sweetness to your taste.

18. Cacao-Avocado Dream

Ingredients
- 1 ripe avocado
- 2 tablespoons cacao powder
- 1 cup unsweetened almond milk
- 1 tablespoon honey (optional)
- A handful of ice cubes

Instructions: Blend all the ingredients until smooth and creamy. Adjust the sweetness and chocolate flavor to your liking.

19. Matcha-Green Tea Booster

Ingredients
- 1 teaspoon matcha green tea powder
- 1 ripe banana

- 1 cup spinach
- 1 cup unsweetened almond milk
- 1 tablespoon honey (optional)

Instructions: Blend all the ingredients together until well combined. Adjust the sweetness and matcha flavor as desired.

20. Watermelon-Cucumber Cooler

Ingredients

- 2 cups watermelon chunks
- 1/2 cucumber
- 1/2 lime (juiced)
- A handful of fresh mint leaves
- A handful of ice cubes

Instructions: Blend all the ingredients until smooth and refreshing. Adjust the lime juice and sweetness to your preference.

21. Acai-Berry Booster

Ingredients

- 1 packet of frozen acai pulp

- 1 cup mixed berries (strawberries, blueberries, raspberries)
- 1 ripe banana
- 1 cup coconut water
- 1 tablespoon chia seeds

Instructions: Blend all the ingredients until smooth and creamy. Adjust the sweetness if desired.

22. Pineapple-Mint Refresher

Ingredients
- 1 cup pineapple chunks
- 1/2 cup fresh mint leaves
- 1/2 lime (juiced)
- 1 cup coconut water
- A handful of ice cubes

Instructions: Blend all the ingredients together until well combined. Adjust the lime juice and mint flavor to your liking.

23. Papaya-Ginger Elixir

Ingredients
- 1 cup ripe papaya chunks

- 1/2 teaspoon ginger powder (or 1-inch piece of fresh ginger)
- 1 cup almond milk
- 1 tablespoon honey (optional)
- A handful of ice cubes

Instructions: Blend all the ingredients until smooth and creamy. Adjust the sweetness and ginger flavor as desired.

24. Spinach-Avocado Green Machine

Ingredients
- 2 cups spinach
- 1/2 ripe avocado
- 1 green apple
- 1 cup unsweetened almond milk
- 1 tablespoon almond butter

Instructions: Blend all the recipes together till smooth and creamy. Adjust the sweetness and consistency to your liking.

25. Blueberry-Walnut Bliss

Ingredients

- 1 cup blueberries
- 1/4 cup walnuts
- 1 cup unsweetened almond milk
- 1 tablespoon honey (optional)
- A handful of ice cubes

Instructions: Blend all the ingredients until well combined. Adjust the sweetness and nuttiness to your preference.

Conclusion

Unlock the Fountain of Youth with "Anti-Aging Juicing and Smoothie Recipes for Beginners." Delve into a world of tantalizing concoctions that defy the hands of time. From the Green Goddess Glow, brimming with vibrant greens and exotic fruits, to the Cocoa Collagen Crush, a decadent elixir of youth, each recipe is a masterpiece crafted to nourish your body from within.

Embrace the power of antioxidants, vitamins, and minerals as they dance on your palate, revitalizing your skin and invigorating your spirit. Join the movement and sip your way to a more youthful you. The secret to eternal vitality awaits within these pages.

www.ingramcontent.com/pod-product-compliance
Lightning Source LLC
Chambersburg PA
CBHW050749250726
48662CB00005B/2097